The Ultimate Keto Diet Dishes Guide

Fast and Delicious Recipes

affordable for Busy People

Otis Fisher

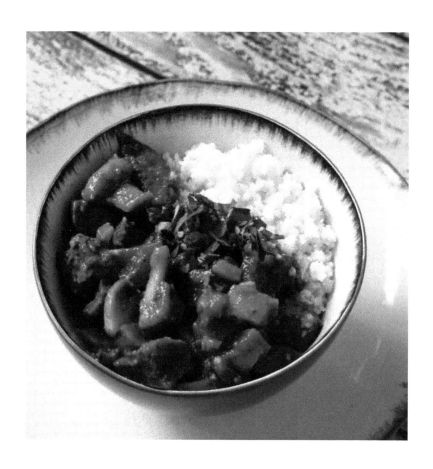

content within this book has been derived from various sources. Please consult a licensed professional before attempting any techniques outlined in this book.

By reading this document, the reader agrees that under no circumstances is the author responsible for any losses, direct or indirect, which are incurred as a result of the use of information contained within this document, including, but not limited to, — errors, omissions, or inaccuracies.

Table of contents

Breakfast Peanut Butter Chaffle

Preparation Time: 7 minutes

Cooking Time: 15 minutes

Servings: 2

Ingredients:

- 1 egg, lightly beaten
- 1/2 tsp. vanilla
- 1 tbsp. Swerve
- 2 tbsp. powdered peanut butter
- 1/2 cup mozzarella cheese, shredded

Directions:

1. Preheat your Chaffle maker.
2. Attach all ingredients into the bowl and mix until well combined.
3. Spray Chaffle maker with Cooking spray.
4. Pour half batter in the hot Chaffle maker and Cooking for 5-7 minutes or until golden brown. Repeat with the remaining batter.
5. Serve and enjoy.

Nutrition:

Calories 80

Fat 4.1 g

Carbohydrates 2.9 g

Sugar 0.g

Protein 7.4 g

Cholesterol 86 mg

Easy Apple Cinnamon Chaffles

Preparation Time: 7 minutes

Cooking Time: 20 minutes

Servings: 3

Ingredients:

- 3 eggs, lightly beaten
- 1 cup mozzarella cheese, shredded
- 1/4 cup apple, chopped
- 1/2 tsp. monk fruit sweetener
- 1 1/2 tsp. cinnamon
- 1/4 tsp. baking powder, gluten-free
- 2 tbsp. coconut flour

Directions:

1. Preheat your Chaffle maker.
2. Attach remaining ingredients and stir until well combined.
3. Spray Chaffle maker with Cooking spray.
4. Pour 1/3 of batter in the hot Chaffle maker and Cooking for minutes or until golden brown. Repeat with the remaining batter.
5. Serve and enjoy.

Nutrition:

Calories 142

Fat 7.4 g

Carbohydrates 9.7 g

Sugar 3 g

Protein 9.g

Cholesterol 169 mg

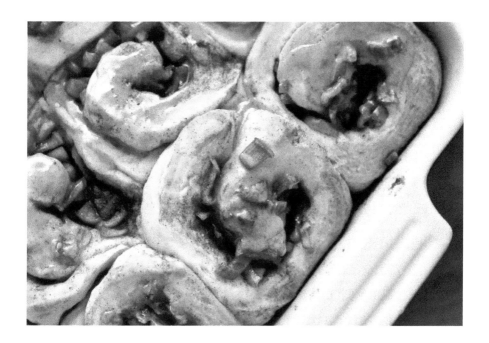

Churro Chaffle

Preparation Time: 7 minutes

Cooking Time: 8 minutes

Servings: 2

Ingredients:

- 1 egg
- 1/2 cup mozzarella cheese, shredded
- 1/2 teaspoon cinnamon
- 2 tablespoons sweetener

Directions:

1. Turn on your Chaffle iron.
2. Beat the egg in a bowl.
3. Stir in the cheese.
4. Set half of the mixture into the Chaffle maker.
5. Cover the Chaffle iron.
6. Cooking for 4 minutes.
7. While waiting, mix the cinnamon and sweetener in a bowl.
8. Open the device and soak the Chaffle in the cinnamon mixture.
9. Repeat the steps with the remaining batter.

Nutrition:

Calories: 123

Total Fat 6.9g

Saturated Fat 2.9g

Cholesterol 171mg

Sodium 147mg

Potassium 64mg

Carbohydrate 5

Crab Chaffle Roll

Preparation Time: 7 minutes

Cooking Time: 10 minutes

Servings: 2

Ingredients:

- Crab Meat: 1 1/2 cup
- Egg: 2
- Mozzarella Cheese: 1 cup (shredded)
- Lemon juice: 2 tsp.
- Kewpie Mayo: 2 tbsp.
- Garlic powder: 1/2 tsp.
- Bay seasoning: 1/2 tsp.

Directions:

1. Cook crab meat if needed
2. In a small mixing bowl, merge crab meat with lemon juice and Kewpie mayo and keep aside
3. In a mixing bowl, beat eggs and add mozzarella cheese to them with garlic powder and bay seasoning
4. Mix them all well and pour to the greasy mini Chaffle maker
5. Cook for at least 4 minutes to get the desired crunch
6. Remove the chaffle from the heat, add the crab mixture in between and fold
7. Make as many chaffles as your mixture and Chaffle maker allow
8. Serve hot and enjoy!

Nutrition:

Calories: 121kcal

Carbohydrates: 3g

Protein: 9g

Fat: 8g

Garlic Lobster Chaffle Roll

Preparation Time: 7 minutes

Cooking Time: 10 minutes

Servings: 2

Ingredients:

For Chaffle:

- Egg: 2
- Mozzarella Cheese: 1 cup (shredded)
- Bay seasoning: 1/2 tsp.
- Garlic powder: 1/4 tsp.

For Lobster Mix:

- Langostino Tails: 1 cup
- Kewpie Mayo: 2 tbsp.
- Garlic powder: 1/2 tsp.
- Lemon juice: 2 tsp.
- Parsley: 1 tsp. (chopped) for garnishing

Directions:

1. Defrost langostino tails
2. In a small mixing bowl, mix langostino tails with lemon juice, garlic powder, and Kewpie mayo; mix properly and keep aside
3. In another mixing bowl, beat eggs and add mozzarella cheese to them with garlic powder and bay seasoning
4. Mix them all well and pour to the greasy mini Chaffle maker

5. Cook for at least 4 minutes to get the desired crunch
6. Remove the chaffle from the heat, add the lobster mixture in between and fold
7. Make as many chaffles as your mixture and Chaffle maker allow
8. Serve hot and enjoy!

Nutrition

Calories 194

Total Fat 13 g

Saturated Fat 7 g

Cholesterol 115 mg

Sodium 789 mg

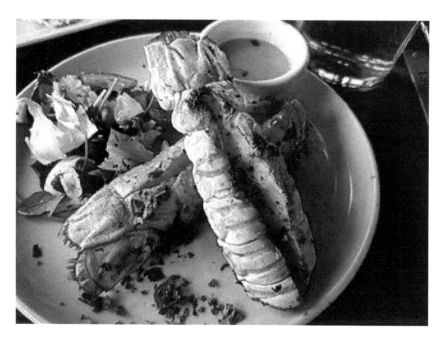

Fried Fish Chaffles

Preparation Time: 7 minutes

Cooking Time: 15 minutes

Servings: 2

Ingredients:

For Chaffle:

- Egg: 2
- Mozzarella Cheese: 1 cup (shredded)
- Bay seasoning: 1/2 tsp.
- Garlic powder: 1/4 tsp.

For Fried Fish:

- Fish boneless: 1 cup
- Garlic powder: 1 tbsp.
- Onion powder: 1 tbsp.
- Salt: 1/4 tsp. or as per your taste
- Black pepper: 1/4 tsp.
- Turmeric: 1/4 tsp.
- Red chili flakes: 1/2 tbsp.
- Butter: 2 tbsp.

Directions:

1. Marinate the fish with all the ingredients of the fried fish except for butter
2. Melt butter in a medium-size frying pan and add the marinated fish

3. Fry from both sides for at least 5 minutes and set aside
4. Preheat a mini Chaffle maker if needed and grease it
5. In a mixing bowl, beat eggs and add all the chaffle ingredients
6. Mix them all well
7. Pour the mixture to the lower plate of the Chaffle maker and spread it evenly to cover the plate properly
8. Close the lid
9. Cook for at least 4 minutes to get the desired crunch
10. Remove the chaffle from the heat and keep aside for around one minute
11. Make as many chaffles as your mixture and Chaffle maker allow
12. Serve hot with the prepared fish

Nutrition:

Calories: 187

Net Carb: 1.8g

Fat: 14.5g

Saturated Fat: 5g

Carbohydrates: 4.

Tuna Melt Chaffle

Preparation Time: 7 minutes

Cooking Time: 20 minutes

Servings: 2

Ingredients:

- Egg: 1
- Mozzarella Cheese: 1/2 cup (shredded)
- Tuna: 3 oz. without water
- Salt: a pinch

Directions:

1. Preheat a mini Chaffle maker if needed and grease it
2. In a mixing bowl, merge all the ingredients well
3. Pour the mixture to the lower plate of the Chaffle maker and spread it evenly to cover the plate properly
4. Close the lid
5. Cook for at least 4 minutes to get the desired crunch
6. Remove the chaffle from the heat and keep aside for around one minute
7. Make as many chaffles as your mixture and Chaffle maker allow
8. Serve hot and enjoy!

Nutrition:

Calories: 170

Fats: 13 g

Carbs: 2 g

Protein: 11 g

Crispy Crab Chaffle

Preparation Time: 7 minutes

Cooking Time: 45 minutes

Servings: 2

Ingredients:

For Chaffle:

- Egg: 1
- Mozzarella Cheese: 1/2 cup (shredded)
- Salt: 1/4 tsp. or as per your taste
- Black pepper: 1/4 tsp.
- Ginger powder: 1 tbsp.

For Crab

- Crab meat: 1 cup
- Butter: 2 tbsp.
- Salt: 1/4 tsp. or as per your taste
- Black pepper: 1/4 tsp.
- Red chili flakes: 1/2 tsp.

Directions:

1. In a frying pan, dissolve butter and fry crab meat for two minutes
2. Add the spices at the end and set aside
3. Mix all the chaffle ingredients well together
4. Pour a thin layer on a preheated Chaffle iron

5. Add prepared crab and pour again more mixture over the top
6. Cook the chaffle for around 5 minutes
7. Make as many chaffles as your mixture and Chaffle maker allow
8. Serve hot with your favorite sauce

Nutrition:

Carbs: 4 g

Fat: 26 g

Protein: 26 g

Calories: 365

Turkey Chaffle Sandwich

Preparation Time: 5 minutes

Cooking Time: 15 minutes

Serving: 4

Ingredients:

Batter

- 4 eggs
- 1/4 cup cream cheese
- 1 cup grated mozzarella cheese
- Salt and pepper to taste
- 1 teaspoon dried dill
- 1/2 teaspoon onion powder
- 1/2 teaspoon garlic powder
- Juicy chicken
- 2 tablespoons butter
- 1 pound chicken breast
- Salt and pepper to taste
- 1 teaspoon dried dill
- 2 tablespoons heavy cream

Other

- 2 tablespoons butter to brush the Chaffle maker
- 4 lettuce leaves to garnish the sandwich
- 4 tomato slices to garnish the sandwich

Directions

1. Preheat the Chaffle maker.
2. Add the eggs, cream cheese, mozzarella cheese, salt and pepper, dried dill, onion powder and garlic powder to a bowl.
3. Mix everything with a fork just until batter forms.
4. Brush the heated Chaffle maker with butter and add a few tablespoons of the batter.
5. Close the lid and Cooking for about 5–7 minutes depending on your Chaffle maker.
6. Meanwhile, heat some butter in a nonstick pan.
7. Season the chicken with salt and pepper and sprinkle with dried dill. Pour the heavy cream on top.
8. Cooking the chicken slices for about 10 minutes or until golden brown.
9. Cut each chaffle in half.
10. On one half add a lettuce leaf, tomato slice, and chicken slice. Cover with the other chaffle half to make a sandwich.
11. Serve and enjoy.

Nutrition

Calories 381

Fat 26.3 g

Carbs 2.5 g

Sugar 1 g,

Protein 32.9 g

Sodium 278 Mg

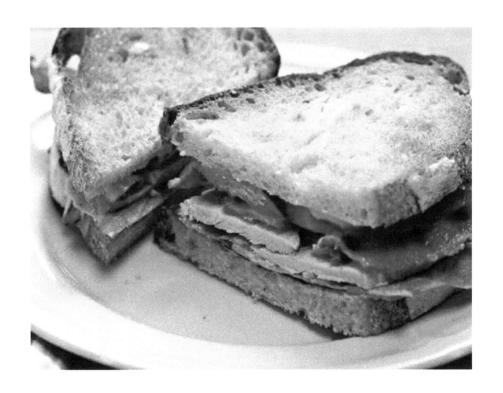

Mozzarella Chicken Jalapeno Chaffle

Preparation Time: 5 minutes

Cooking Time: 8 minutes

Serving: 2

Ingredients:

Batter

- 1/2 pound ground chicken
- 4 eggs
- 1 cup grated mozzarella cheese
- 2 tablespoons sour cream
- 1 green jalapeno, chopped
- Salt and pepper to taste
- 1 teaspoon dried oregano
- 1/2 teaspoon dried garlic

Other

- 2 tablespoons butter to brush the Chaffle maker
- 1/4 cup sour cream to garnish
- 1 green jalapeno, diced, to garnish

Directions

1. Preheat the Chaffle maker.
2. Add the ground chicken, eggs, mozzarella cheese, sour cream, chopped jalapeno, salt and pepper, dried oregano and dried garlic to a bowl.
3. Mix everything until batter forms.

4. Brush the heated Chaffle maker with butter and add a few tablespoons of the batter.
5. Close the lid and Cooking for about 8–10 minutes depending on your Chaffle maker.
6. Serve with a tablespoon of sour cream and sliced jalapeno on top.

Nutrition

Calories 284

Fat 19.4 G

Carbs 2.2 G

Sugar 0.6 G,

Protein 24.7 G

Sodium 204 Mg

Turkey BBQ Sauce Chaffle

Preparation Time: 5 minutes

Cooking Time: 10 minutes

Serving: 4

Ingredients:

Batter

- 1/2 pound ground turkey meat
- 3 eggs
- 1 cup grated Swiss cheese
- 1/4 cup cream cheese
- 1/4 cup BBQ sauce
- 1 teaspoon dried oregano
- Salt and pepper to taste
- 2 cloves garlic, minced

Other

- 2 tablespoons butter to brush the Chaffle maker
- 1/4 cup BBQ sauce for serving
- 2 tablespoons freshly chopped parsley for garnish

Directions

1. Preheat the Chaffle maker.
2. Add the ground turkey, eggs, grated Swiss cheese, cream cheese, BBQ sauce, dried oregano, salt and pepper, and minced garlic to a bowl.
3. Mix everything until combined and batter forms.

4. Brush the heated Chaffle maker with butter and add a few tablespoons of the batter.
5. Close the lid and Cooking for about 8–10 minutes depending on your Chaffle maker.
6. Serve each chaffle with a tablespoon of BBQ sauce and a sprinkle of freshly chopped parsley.

Nutrition

Calories 365

Fat 23.7 g

Carbs 13.7 g

Sugar 8.8 g,

Protein 23.5 g

Sodium 595 mg

Protein 27.4 g

Sodium 291 Mg

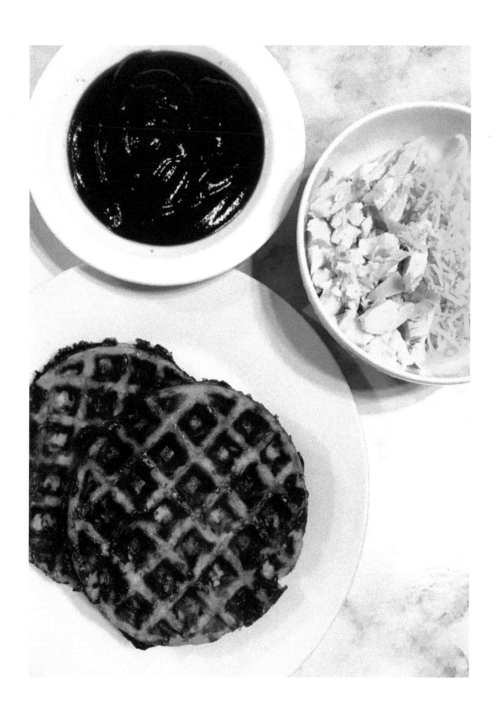

Beef and Sour Cream Chaffle

Preparation Time: 5 minutes

Cooking Time: 20 minutes

Serving: 4

Ingredients:

Batter

- 4 eggs
- 2 cups grated mozzarella cheese
- 3 tablespoons coconut flour
- 3 tablespoons almond flour
- 2 teaspoons baking powder
- Salt and pepper to taste
- 1 tablespoon freshly chopped parsley
- Seasoned beef
- 1 pound beef tenderloin
- Salt and pepper to taste
- 2 tablespoons olive oil
- 1 tablespoon Dijon mustard

Other

- 2 tablespoons olive oil to brush the Chaffle maker
- 1/4 cup sour cream for garnish
- 2 tablespoons freshly chopped spring onion for garnish

Directions

1. Preheat the Chaffle maker.
2. Add the eggs, grated mozzarella cheese, coconut flour, almond flour, baking powder, salt and pepper and freshly chopped parsley to a bowl.
3. Mix until just combined and batter forms.
4. Brush the heated Chaffle maker with olive oil and add a few tablespoons of the batter.
5. Close the lid and Cooking for about 5–7 minutes depending on your Chaffle maker.
6. Meanwhile, heat the olive oil in a nonstick pan over medium heat.
7. Season the beef tenderloin with salt and pepper and spread the whole piece of beef tenderloin with Dijon mustard.
8. Cooking on each side for about 4–5 minutes.
9. Serve each chaffle with sour cream and slices of the cooked beef tenderloin.
10. Garnish with freshly chopped spring onion.
11. Serve and enjoy.

Nutrition

Calories 543

Fat 37 g

Carbs 7.9 g

Sugar 0.5 g

Protein 44.9 g

Sodium 269 Mg

Beef Chaffle Sandwich Recipe

Preparation Time: 5 minutes

Cooking Time: 15 minutes

Serving: 4

Ingredients:

Batter

- 3 eggs
- 2 cups grated mozzarella cheese
- 1/4 cup cream cheese
- Salt and pepper to taste
- 1 teaspoon Italian seasoning

Beef

- 2 tablespoons butter
- 1 pound beef tenderloin
- Salt and pepper to taste
- 2 teaspoons Dijon mustard
- 1 teaspoon dried paprika

Other

- 2 tablespoons Cooking spray to brush the Chaffle maker
- 4 lettuce leaves for serving
- 4 tomato slices for serving
- 4 leaves fresh basil

Directions

Preheat the Chaffle maker.

1. Add the eggs, grated mozzarella cheese, salt and pepper and Italian seasoning to a bowl.
2. Mix until combined and batter forms.
3. Brush the heated Chaffle maker with Cooking spray and add a few tablespoons of the batter.
4. Close the lid and Cooking for about 5–7 minutes depending on your Chaffle maker.
5. Meanwhile, melt and heat the butter in a nonstick frying pan.
6. Season the beef loin with salt and pepper, brush it with Dijon mustard, and sprinkle some dried paprika on top.
7. Cooking the beef on each side for about 5 minutes.
8. Thinly slice the beef and assemble the chaffle sandwiches.
9. Cut each chaffle in half and on one half place a lettuce leaf, tomato slice, basil leaf, and some sliced beef.
10. Cover with the other chaffle half and serve.

Nutrition

Calories 477

Fat 32.8g

Carbs 2.3 g

Sugar 0.9 g,

Protein 42.2 g

Sodium 299 Mg

Beef Meatballs on a Chaffle

Preparation Time: 5 minutes

Cooking Time: 20 minutes

Serving: 4

Ingredients:

Batter

- 4 eggs
- 21/2 cups grated gouda cheese
- 1/4 cup heavy cream
- Salt and pepper to taste
- 1 spring onion, finely chopped

Beef meatballs

- 1 pound ground beef
- Salt and pepper to taste
- 2 teaspoons Dijon mustard
- 1 spring onion, finely chopped
- 5 tablespoons almond flour
- 2 tablespoons butter

Other

- 2 tablespoons Cooking spray to brush the Chaffle maker
- 2 tablespoons freshly chopped parsley

Directions

1. Preheat the Chaffle maker.

2. Add the eggs, grated gouda cheese, heavy cream, salt and pepper and finely chopped spring onion to a bowl.

3. Mix until combined and batter forms.

4. Brush the heated Chaffle maker with Cooking spray and add a few tablespoons of the batter.

5. Close the lid and Cooking for about 5–7 minutes depending on your Chaffle maker.

6. Meanwhile, mix the ground beef meat, salt and pepper, Dijon mustard, chopped spring onion and almond flour in a large bowl.

7. Form small meatballs with your hands.

8. Warmth the butter in a nonstick frying pan and Cooking the beef meatballs for about 3–4 minutes on each side.

9. Serve each chaffle with a couple of meatballs and some freshly chopped parsley on top.

Nutrition

Calories 670

Fat 47.4g

Carbs 4.6 g

Sugar 1.7 g,

Protein 54.9 g

Sodium 622 Mg

Beef Chaffle Taco

Preparation Time: 5 minutes

Cooking Time: 15 minutes

Serving: 4

Ingredients:

Batter

- 4 eggs
- 2 cups grated cheddar cheese
- 1/4 cup heavy cream
- Salt and pepper to taste
- 1/4 cup almond flour
- 2 teaspoons baking powder

Beef

- 2 tablespoons butter
- 1/2 onion, diced
- 1 pound ground beef
- Salt and pepper to taste
- 1 teaspoon dried oregano
- 1 tablespoon sugar-free ketchup

Other

- 2 tablespoons Cooking spray to brush the Chaffle maker
- 2 tablespoons freshly chopped parsley

Directions

1. Preheat the Chaffle maker.
2. Add the eggs, grated cheddar cheese, heavy cream, salt and pepper, almond flour and baking powder to a bowl.
3. Brush the heated Chaffle maker with Cooking spray and add a few tablespoons of the batter.
4. Close the lid and Cooking for about 5–7 minutes depending on your Chaffle maker.
5. Once the chaffle is ready, place it in a napkin holder to harden into the shape of a taco as it cools.
6. Meanwhile, melt and heat the butter in a nonstick frying pan and start Cooking the diced onion.
7. Once the onion is tender, add the ground beef. Season with salt and pepper and dried oregano and stir in the sugar-free ketchup.
8. Cooking for about 7 minutes.
9. Serve the Cooked ground meat in each taco chaffle sprinkled with some freshly chopped parsley.

Nutrition

Calories 719

Fat 51.7 g

Carbs 7.3 g

Sugar 1.3 g,

Protein 56.1 g

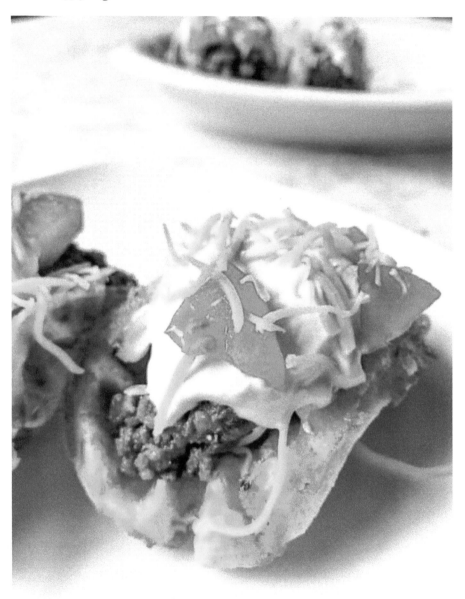

Beef Meatza Chaffle

Preparation Time: 5 minutes

Cooking Time: 20 minutes

Serving: 4

Ingredients:

- Meatza chaffle batter
- 1/2 pound ground beef
- 4 eggs
- 2 cups grated cheddar cheese
- Salt and pepper to taste
- 1 teaspoon Italian seasoning
- 2 tablespoons tomato sauce

Other

- 2 tablespoons Cooking spray to brush the Chaffle maker
- 1/4 cup tomato sauce for serving
- 2 tablespoons freshly chopped basil for serving

Directions

Preheat the Chaffle maker.

1. Add the ground beef, eggs, grated cheddar cheese, salt and pepper, Italian seasoning and tomato sauce to a bowl.
2. Mix until everything is fully combined.
3. Brush the heated Chaffle maker with Cooking spray and add a few tablespoons of the batter.

4. Close the lid and Cooking for about 7–10 minutes depending on your Chaffle maker.

5. Serve with tomato sauce and freshly chopped basil on top.

Nutrition

Calories 470

Fat 34.6 g

Carbs 2.5 g

Sugar 1.7 g,

Protein 36.5

Sodium 581 Mg

Beef Chaffle Tower

Preparation Time: 5 minutes

Cooking Time: 15 minutes

Serving: 4

Ingredients:

Batter

- 4 eggs
- 2 cups grated mozzarella cheese
- Salt and pepper to taste
- 2 tablespoons almond flour
- 1 teaspoon Italian seasoning

Beef

- 2 tablespoons butter
- 1 pound beef tenderloin
- Salt and pepper to taste
- 1 teaspoon chili flakes

Other

- 2 tablespoons Cooking spray to brush the Chaffle maker

Directions

1. Preheat the Chaffle maker.
2. Add the eggs, grated mozzarella cheese, salt and pepper, almond flour and Italian seasoning to a bowl.
3. Mix until everything is fully combined.

4. Brush the heated Chaffle maker with Cooking spray and add a few tablespoons of the batter.
5. Close the lid and Cooking for about 5–7 minutes depending on your Chaffle maker.
6. Meanwhile, heat the butter in a nonstick frying pan and season the beef tenderloin with salt and pepper and chili flakes.
7. Cooking the beef tenderloin for about 5–7 minutes on each side.
8. When serving, assemble the chaffle tower by placing one chaffle on a plate, a layer of diced beef tenderloin, another chaffle, another layer of beef, and so on until you finish with the Chaffles and beef.
9. Serve and enjoy.

Nutrition

Calories 412

Fat 25 g

Carbs 1.8 g

Sugar 0.5 g,

Protein 43.2 g

Sodium 256 Mg

Keto Pork Tzatziki Chaffle

Preparation Time: 5 minutes

Cooking Time: 25 minutes

Serving: 4

Ingredients:

- 4 eggs
- 2 cups grated provolone cheese
- Salt and pepper to taste
- 1 teaspoon dried rosemary
- 1 teaspoon dried oregano
- Pork loin
- 2 tablespoons olive oil
- 1 pound pork tenderloin
- Salt and pepper to taste
- Tzatziki sauce
- 1 cup sour cream
- Salt and pepper to taste
- 1 cucumber, peeled and diced
- 1 teaspoon garlic powder
- 1 teaspoon dried dill
- 2 tablespoons butter to brush the Chaffle maker

Directions

1. Preheat the Chaffle maker.

2. Add the eggs, grated provolone cheese, dried rosemary, and dried oregano to a bowl. Season with salt and pepper to taste.
3. Mix until combined.
4. Brush the heated Chaffle maker with butter and add a few tablespoons of the batter.
5. Secure the lid and Cook for about 5—7 minutes depending on your Chaffle maker.
6. Meanwhile, heat the olive oil in a nonstick frying pan. Generously season the pork tenderloin with salt and pepper and Cook it for about 7 minutes on each side.
7. Mix the sour cream, salt and pepper, diced cucumber, garlic powder and dried dill in a bowl.
8. Serve each chaffle with a few tablespoons of tzatziki sauce and slices of pork tenderloin.

Nutrition

Calories 700

Fat 50.9 g

Carbs 6 g

Sugar 1.5 g

Protein 54.4 g

Sodium 777 Mg

Pecan Pie Cake Chaffle

Preparation Time: 15 minutes

Cooking Time: 25 minutes

Servings: 2

Ingredients:

For Pecan Pie Chaffle:

- Egg: 1
- Cream cheese: 2 tbsp.
- Maple extract: 1/2 tbsp.
- Almond flour: 4 tbsp.
- Serkin Gold: 1 tbsp.
- Baking powder: 1/2 tbsp.
- Pecan: 2 tbsp. chopped
- Heavy whipping cream: 1 tbsp.

For Pecan Pie Filling:

- Butter: 2 tbsp.
- Serkin Gold: 1 tbsp.
- Pecan: 2 tbsp. chopped
- Heavy whipping cream: 2 tbsp.
- Maple syrup: 2 tbsp.
- Egg yolk: 2 large
- Salt: a pinch

Directions:

1. In a small saucepan, add sweetener, butter, syrups, and heavy whipping cream and use a low flame to heat
2. Mix all the ingredients well together
3. Remove from heat and add egg yolks and mix
4. Now put it on heat again and stir
5. Add pecan and salt to the mixture and let it simmer
6. It will thicken then detach from heat and let it rest
7. For the chaffles, add all the ingredients except pecans and blend
8. Now add pecan with a spoon
9. Preheat a mini Chaffle maker if needed and grease it
10. Pour the mixture to the lower plate of the Chaffle maker and spread it evenly to cover the plate properly and close the lid
11. Cooking for at least 4 minutes to get the desired crunch
12. Remove the chaffle from the heat and keep aside for around one minute
13. Make as many chaffles as your mixture and Chaffle maker allow
14. Add 1/3 the previously prepare pecan pie filling to the chaffle and arrange like a cake

Nutrition:

Calories 141

Protein 10 g

Carbohydrates 15 g

Fat 0 g

Sodium 113 mg

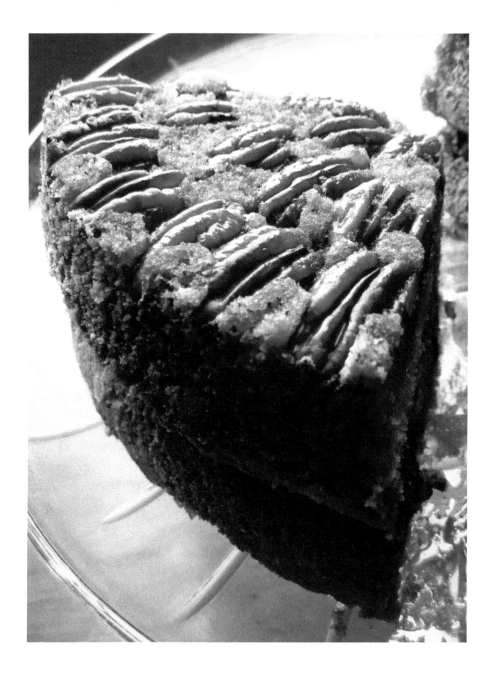

German Chocolate Chaffle Cake

Preparation Time: 5 minutes

Cooking Time: 10 minutes

Servings: 2

Ingredients:

For Chocolate Chaffle:

- Egg: 1
- Cream cheese: 2 tbsp.
- Powdered sweetener: 1 tbsp.
- Vanilla extract: 1/2 tbsp.
- Instant coffee powder: 1/4 tsp.
- Almond flour: 1 tbsp.
- Cocoa powder: 1 tbsp. (unsweetened)

For Filling:

- Egg Yolk: 1
- Heavy cream: 1/4 cup
- Butter: 1 tbsp.
- Powdered sweetener: 2 tbsp.
- Caramel: 1/2 tsp.
- Coconut flakes: 1/4 cup
- Coconut flour: 1 tsp.
- Pecans: 1/4 cups chopped

Directions:

1. Preheat a mini Chaffle maker if needed and grease it

2. In a mixing bowl, beat eggs and add the remaining chaffle ingredients
3. Mix them all well
4. Pour the mixture to the lower plate of the Chaffle maker and spread it evenly to cover the plate properly and close the lid
5. Cooking for at least 4 minutes to get the desired crunch
6. Remove the chaffle from the heat and let them cool completely
7. Make as many chaffles as your mixture and Chaffle maker allow
8. In a small pan, mix heavy cream, egg yolk, sweetener, and butter at low heat for around 5 minutes
9. Remove from heat and add the remaining ingredients to make the filling
10. Stack chaffles on one another and add filling in between to enjoy the cake

Nutrition:

Calories 147

Fat 11.5 g

Protein 9.8 g

Almond Chocolate Chaffle Cake

Preparation Time: 5 minutes

Cooking Time: 10 minutes

Servings: 2

Ingredients:

For Chocolate Chaffle:

Egg: 1

- Cream cheese: 2 tbsp.
- Powdered sweetener: 1 tbsp.
- Vanilla extract: 1/2 tbsp.
- Instant coffee powder: 1/4 tsp.
- Almond flour: 1 tbsp.
- Cocoa powder: 1 tbsp. (unsweetened)

For Coconut Filling:

- Melted Coconut Oil: 1 1/2 tbsp.
- Heavy cream: 1 tbsp.
- Cream cheese: 4 tbsp.
- Powdered sweetener: 1 tbsp.
- Vanilla extract: 1/2 tbsp.
- Coconut: 1/4 cup finely shredded
- Whole almonds: 14

Directions:

1. Preheat a mini Chaffle maker if needed and grease it
2. In a mixing bowl, add all the chaffle ingredients

3. Mix them all well
4. Pour the mixture to the lower plate of the Chaffle maker and spread it evenly to cover the plate properly
5. Close the lid
6. Cooking for at least 4 minutes to get the desired crunch
7. Remove the chaffle from the heat and keep aside for around one minute
8. Make as many chaffles as your mixture and Chaffle maker allow
9. Except for almond, add all the filling ingredients in a bowl and mix well
10. Spread the filling on the chaffle and spread almonds on top with another chaffle at almonds stack the chaffles and fillings like a cake and enjoy

Nutrition

Calories 238

Fat 18.4g

Protein 14.3g

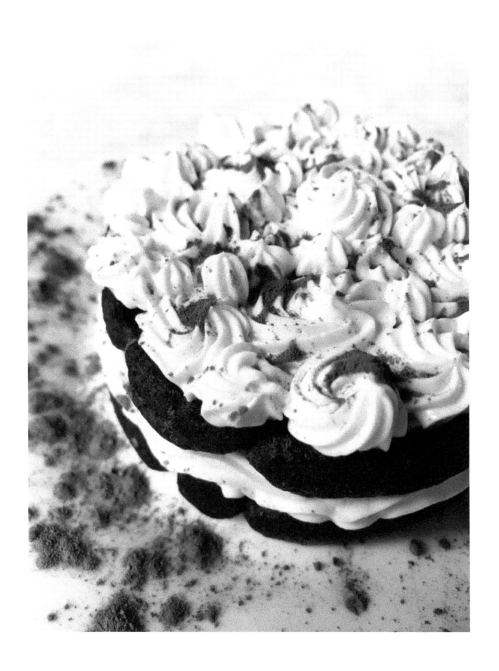

Carrot Cake Chaffle

Preparation Time: 10 minutes

Cooking Time: 15 minutes

Servings: 2

Ingredients:

For Carrot Chaffle Cake:

- Carrot: 1/2 cup (shredded)
- Egg: 1
- Heavy whipping cream: 2 tbsp.
- Butter: 2 tbsp. (melted)
- Powdered sweetener: 2 tbsp.
- Walnuts: 1 tbsp. (chopped)
- Almond flour: 3/4 cup
- Cinnamon powder: 2 tsp.
- Baking powder: 1 tsp.
- Pumpkin sauce: 1 tsp.

For Cream Cheese Frosting:

- Cream cheese: 1/2 cup
- Heavy whipping cream: 2 tbsp.
- Vanilla extract: 1 tsp.
- Powdered sweetener: 1/4 cup

Directions:

1. Merge all the ingredients together one by one until they form a uniform consistency

2. Preheat a mini Chaffle maker if needed and grease it
3. Pour the mixture to the lower plate of the Chaffle maker
4. Close the lid
5. Cooking for at least 4 minutes to get the desired crunch
6. Prepare frosting by combining all the ingredients of the cream cheese frosting using a hand mixer
7. Remove the chaffle from the heat and keep aside for around a few minutes
8. Make as many chaffles as your mixture and Chaffle maker allow
9. Stack the chaffles with frosting in between in such a way that it gives the look of a cake

Nutrition:

Calories 555

Total Fat 21.5g

Saturated Fat 3.5g

Cholesterol 117mg

Sodium 654mg

Peanut Butter Keto Chaffle Cake

Preparation Time: 5 minutes

Cooking Time: 10 minutes

Servings: 2

Ingredients:

For Chaffles:

- Egg: 1
- Peanut Butter:: 2 tbsp. (sugar-free)
- Monk fruit: 2 tbsp.
- Baking powder: 1/4 tsp.
- Peanut butter extract: 1/4 tsp.
- Heavy whipping cream: 1 tsp.

For Peanut Butter Frosting:

- Monk fruit: 2 tsp.
- Cream cheese: 2 tbsp.
- Butter: 1 tbsp.
- Peanut butter: 1 tbsp. (sugar-free)
- Vanilla: 1/4 tsp.

Directions:

1. Preheat a mini Chaffle maker if needed and grease it
2. In a mixing bowl, beat eggs and add all the chaffle ingredients
3. Merge them all well and pour the mixture to the lower plate of the Chaffle maker

4. Close the lid
5. Cooking for at least 4 minutes to get the desired crunch
6. Remove the chaffle from the heat and keep aside for around a few minutes
7. Make as many chaffles as your mixture and Chaffle maker allow
8. In a separate bowl, add all the frosting ingredients and whisk well to give it a uniform consistency
9. Assemble chaffles in a way that in between two chaffles you put the frosting and make the cake

Nutrition:

Calories: 127

Net Carb: 2gFat: 9g

Saturated Fat: 5.3g

Carbohydrates: 2.7g

Dietary Fiber: 0.7g

Strawberry Shortcake Chaffle

Preparation Time: 5 minutes

Cooking Time: 10 minutes

Servings: 2

Ingredients:

- Egg: 1
- Heavy Whipping Cream: 1 tbsp.
- Any non-sugar sweetener: 2 tbsp.
- Coconut Flour: 1 tsp.
- Cake batter extract: 1/2 tsp.
- Baking powder: 1/4 tsp.
- Strawberry: 4 or as per your taste

Directions:

1. Preheat a mini Chaffle maker if needed and grease it
2. In a mixing bowl, beat eggs and add non-sugar sweetener, coconut flour, baking powder, and cake batter extract
3. Merge them all well and pour the mixture to the lower plate of the Chaffle maker
4. Close the lid
5. Cooking for at least 4 minutes to get the desired crunch
6. Remove the chaffle from the heat and keep aside for around two minutes
7. Make as many chaffles as your mixture and Chaffle maker allow
8. Serve with whipped cream and strawberries on top

Nutrition:

Calories 334

Fat 12.1g

Protein 48.2g

Italian Cream Chaffle Cake

Preparation Time: 8 minutes

Cooking Time: 12 minutes

Servings: 3

Ingredients:

For Chaffle:

- Egg: 4
- Mozzarella Cheese: 1/2 cup
- Almond flour: 1 tbsp.
- Coconut flour: 4 tbsp.
- Monk fruit sweetener: 1 tbsp.
- Vanilla extract: 1 tsp.
- Baking powder: 1 1/2 tsp.
- Cinnamon powder: 1/2 tsp.
- Butter: 1 tbsp. (melted)
- Coconut: 1 tsp. (shredded)
- Walnuts: 1 tsp. (chopped)
- For Italian Cream Frosting:
- Cream cheese: 4 tbsp.
- Butter: 2 tbsp.
- Vanilla: 1/2 tsp.
- Monk fruit sweetener: 2 tbs.

Directions:

1. Blend eggs, cream cheese, sweetener, vanilla, coconut flour, melted butter, almond flour, and baking powder
2. Make the mixture creamy
3. Preheat a mini Chaffle maker if needed and grease it
4. Pour the mixture to the lower plate of the Chaffle maker
5. Close the lid
6. Cooking for at least 4 minutes to get the desired crunch
7. Remove the chaffle from the heat and keep aside to cool it
8. Make as many chaffles as your mixture and Chaffle maker allow
9. Garnish with shredded coconut and chopped walnuts

Nutrition:

Calories: 71

Net Carb: 0.7g

Fat: 4.2g

Carbohydrates: 0.8g

Dietary Fiber: 0.1g

Banana Cake Pudding Chaffle

Preparation Time: 10 minutes

Cooking Time: 1 hour

Servings: 2

Ingredients:

For Banana Chaffle:

- Cream cheese: 2 tbsp.
- Banana extract: 1 tsp.
- Mozzarella cheese: 1/4 cup
- Egg: 1
- Sweetener: 2 tbsp.
- Almond flour: 4 tbsp.
- Baking powder: 1 tsp.

For Banana Pudding:

- Egg yolk: 1 large
- Powdered sweetener: 3 tbsp.
- Xanthan gum: 1/2 tsp.
- Heavy whipping cream: 1/2 cup
- Banana extract: 1/2 tsp.
- Salt: a pinch

Directions:

1. In a pan, add powdered sweetener, heavy cream, and egg yolk and whisk continuously so the mixture thickens
2. Simmer for a minute only

3. Add xanthan gum to the mixture and whisk again
4. Remove the pan from heat and add banana extract and salt and mix them all well
5. Shift the mixture to a glass dish and refrigerate the pudding
6. Preheat a mini Chaffle maker if needed and grease it
7. In a mixing bowl, add all the chaffle ingredients
8. Merge them all well and pour the mixture to the lower plate of the Chaffle maker
9. Close the lid
10. Cooking for at least 5 minutes to get the desired crunch
11. Remove the chaffle from the heat and keep aside for around a few minutes
12. Stack chaffles and pudding one by one to form a cake

Nutrition:

Calories 156

Protein 14 g,

Fat 0 g

Cholesterol 0 mg

Cream Coconut Chaffle Cake

Preparation Time: 20 minutes

Cooking Time: 1 hour 20 minutes (depends on your refrigerator)

Servings: 2

Ingredients:

For Chaffles:

- Egg: 2
- Powdered sweetener: 2 tbsp.
- Cream cheese: 2 tbsp.
- Vanilla extract: 1/2 tsp.
- Butter: 1 tbsp. (melted)
- Coconut: 2 tbsp. (shredded)
- Coconut extract: 1/2 tsp.

For Filling:

- Coconut: 1/4 cup (shredded)
- Butter: 2 tsp.
- Monk fruit sweetener: 2 tbsp.
- Xanthan gum: 1/4 tsp.
- Salt: a pinch
- Egg yolks: 2
- Almond: 1/3 cup unsweetened
- Coconut milk: 1/3 cup

For Garnishing:

- Whipped Cream: as per your taste

- Coconut: 1 tbsp. (shredded)

Directions:

1. Preheat a mini Chaffle maker if needed and grease it
2. In a mixing bowl, add all the chaffle ingredients
3. Merge them all well and pour the mixture to the lower plate of the Chaffle maker
4. Close the lid
5. Cooking for at least 4 minutes to get the desired crunch
6. Remove the chaffle from the heat and keep aside for around a few minutes
7. Make as many chaffles as your mixture and Chaffle maker allow
8. For the filling, in a small pan, Cooking almond milk and coconut together on medium heat in such way that it only steams but doesn't boil
9. In another bowl, lightly whish egg yolks and add milk to it continuously
10. Heat the mixture so it thickens, again it must not boil
11. Add sweetener and whisk while adding Xanthan Gum bit by bit
12. Remove from heat and mix all the other ingredients
13. Mix well and refrigerate; the mixture will further thicken when cool
14. Assemble the prepare chaffles and cream on top of one another to make the cake-like shape
15. Garnish with coconuts and whipped cream at the end

Nutrition:

Calories: 74

Fat: 2 g

Protein: 4 g,

Carbohydrates: 10 g

Fiber: 0.2 g

Lemon Chaffle Cake

Preparation Time: 40 minutes

Cooking Time: 20 minutes

Servings: 2

Ingredients:

For Chaffles:

- Egg: 2
- Powdered sweetener: 1 tbsp.
- Cream cheese: 4 tbsp.
- Butter: 2 tbsp. (melted)
- Coconut flour: 2 tsp.
- Baking powder: 1 tsp.
- Lemon extract: 1/2 tsp.
- Cake batter extract: 20 drops

For Frosting:

- Heavy whipping cream: 1/2 cup
- Monk fruit sweetener: 1 tbsp.
- Lemon extract: 1/4 tsp.

Directions:

1. Preheat a mini Chaffle maker if needed and grease it
2. In a blender, attach all the chaffle ingredients and blend
3. Pour the mixture to the lower plate of the Chaffle maker and spread it evenly to cover the plate properly
4. Close the lid

5. Cooking for at least 4 minutes to get the desired crunch
6. Remove the chaffle from the heat and keep aside
7. Make as many chaffles as your mixture and Chaffle maker allow
8. Prepare the frosting by whisking all the frosting ingredients till it thickens and attains uniform consistency
9. When all the chaffles cool down, arrange in the form of cake by adding frosting in between

Nutrition:

Calories 552

Fats 28.37g

Protein 59.8g

Creamy Veggie Chaffle

Preparation Time: 5 minutes

Cooking Time: 8 minutes

Servings: 2 chaffles

Ingredients:

- 1 egg
- 1/2 cup zucchini, grated
- 1/2 cup mozzarella cheese, shredded
- 1/2 tbsp. onion, minced
- 1/2 tbsp. tomato, diced
- 1 garlic clove, minced
- Fresh dill, chopped
- A pinch of salt
- 2 tbsp. softened cream cheese for topping

Directions:

1. Heat up the Chaffle maker.
2. Set eggs in bowl and whisk in zucchini, onions, garlic, herbs, tomatoes and most of the cheese.
3. Set half of the batter into the Chaffle maker and Cooking for 4 minutes until brown. Do it again with the rest of the batter to make another chaffle.
4. Let cool for 3 minutes to let chaffles get crispy.
5. Spread the chaffle with softened cream cheese.
6. Serve and enjoy!

Nutrition:

Calories: 103

Net Carb: 2.4g

Fat: 6.6g

Carbohydrates: 2.9g

Dietary Fiber: 0.5g

Tasty Scallion Chaffle

Preparation Time: 5 minutes

Cooking Time: 8 minutes

Servings: 2 chaffles

Ingredients for chaffles:

- 1 large egg, beaten
- 1/2 cup of mozzarella cheese, shredded
- 2 tbsp. almond flour
- 1/4 tsp. baking powder
- 1 tbsp. scallion browned and chopped
- 1 tsp. fresh basil
- A pinch of salt

Ingredients for topping:

- 2 slices Gruyère cheese
- 2 slices deli ham

Directions:

1. Heat up the Chaffle maker.
2. Attach all the ingredients to a small mixing bowl and combine well.
3. Set half of the batter into the Chaffle maker and Cooking for 4 minutes until brown.
4. Let cool for 3 minutes to let chaffles get crispy.
5. Top each chaffle with a slice of Gruyère and a slice of deli ham.
6. Serve and enjoy!

Nutrition:

Calories: 145g

Net Carb: 0.5g

Fat: 11.6g

Carbohydrates: 0.5g

Dietary Fiber: 0g

Mayo and Vegetables Chaffle

Preparation Time: 5 minutes

Cooking Time: 16 minutes

Servings: 4

Ingredients for chaffles:

- 2 large eggs, beaten
- 2 tbsp. keto mayonnaise
- 1 tbsp. almond flour
- 1/4 tsp. baking powder
- 1 tbsp. cream cheese
- A pinch of salt and pepper

Ingredients for topping:

- Lettuce leaves
- 1 tomato sliced
- 1 onion, sliced and browned
- 4-6 slices of grilled zucchini
- 4 slices of grilled eggplant

Directions:

1. Heat up the Chaffle maker.
2. Attach all the ingredients to a small mixing bowl and stir until well combined.
3. Pour 1/4 of the batter into the Chaffle maker and Cooking for 4 minutes until brown.
4. Let cool for 3 minutes to let chaffles get crispy.

5. Garnish the chaffles with lettuce, tomato, onions, zucchini and eggplant slices.
6. Serve warm and enjoy!

Nutrition:

Calories: 98

Net Carb: 1.4g

Fat: 7.1g

Carbohydrates: 2.2g

Eggplant and Bacon Chaffle

Preparation Time: 5 minutes

Cooking Time: 8 minutes

Servings: 2

Ingredients for chaffles:

- 1 egg, beaten
- 1/2 cup shredded mozzarella cheese
- 2 tbsp. bacon bits
- A pinch of salt

Ingredients for topping:

- 2-4 slices of grilled eggplants, very thin
- 2 tbsp. keto mayonnaise
- Fresh parsley to taste

Directions:

1. Heat up the Chaffle maker.
2. Attach all the ingredients to a small mixing bowl and combine well.
3. Set half of the batter into the Chaffle maker and Cooking for 4 minutes until brown.
4. Spread the chaffle with mayonnaise, top with a slice of grilled eggplant and season with fresh minced parsley.
5. Serve and enjoy!

Nutrition:

Calories: 34

Net Carb: 2.4g

Fat: 5.1g

Carbohydrates: 3 g

Creamy Turnip Chaffle

Preparation Time: 5 minutes

Cooking Time: 8 minutes

Servings: 2

Ingredients

For chaffle:

- 1 egg, beaten
- 1/2 cup Monterey Jack cheese, shredded
- 1 turnip, cooked and mashed
- 2 tbsp. ham diced

For topping:

- 2 tbsp. softened cream cheese
- 1 tbsp. fresh basil, chopped

Directions:

1. Heat up the Chaffle maker.
2. Add all the chaffles ingredients to a small mixing bowl and stir until well combined.
3. Set half of the batter into the Chaffle maker and Cooking for 4 minutes until golden brown.
4. Spread the chaffle with cream cheese and season with fresh basil.
5. Serve and enjoy!

Nutrition

Calories: 136 kcal

Cholesterol: 104 mg

Carbohydrates: 2 g

Protein: 10 g

Ground Beef Chaffle

Preparation Time: 4 minutes

Cooking Time: 20 minutes

Servings: 2

Ingredients

For chaffles:

- 1 egg, beaten
- 1/2 cup shredded cheddar cheese
- 1/2 tbsp. fresh basil, finely chopped
- A pinch of salt

For beef:

- 1 tsp. olive oil
- 2 cups ground beef
- 1/2 tsp. garlic powder
- 1 scallion, chopped
- 2 tsp. butter for topping
- 2-3 spinach leaves for topping

Directions:

For chaffles:

1. Heat up the Chaffle maker.
2. Add egg, shredded cheddar cheese, a pinch of salt and basil to a small mixing bowl and combine well.
3. Set half of the batter into the Chaffle maker and Cooking for 4 minutes until brown.

79

Directions for beef:

1. In a saucepan over medium heat Cooking the ground beef in olive oil. Season with salt and pepper if needed and add scallion. Stir occasionally and Cooking until the meat is browned.
2. Instruction for topping:
3. Spread the chaffle with butter, garnish with spinach leaves and beef.
4. Serve and enjoy!

Nutrition:

Cal 215

Net Carbs 4g

Fat 15g

Protein 12g

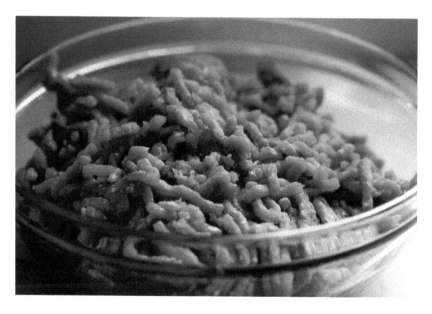

Parsley and Hard-Boiled Egg Chaffle

Preparation Time: 4 minutes

Cooking Time: 8 minutes

Servings: 2

Ingredients

For chaffles:

- 1 large egg, beaten
- 1/2 cup of mozzarella cheese, shredded
- 2 tbsp. almond flour
- 1/4 tsp. baking powder

For topping:

- 1 tbsp. chopped fresh parsley
- 2 tbsp. keto mayonnaise
- 1 hard-boiled egg, thin sliced

Directions:

1. Heat up the Chaffle maker.
2. Add all the chaffles ingredients in a small mixing bowl and combine well.
3. Set half of the batter into the Chaffle maker and Cooking for 4 minutes until brown.
4. Let cool for 3 minutes to let chaffles get crispy.
5. Spread the chaffle with mayonnaise, garnish with a few slices of hard-boiled egg and sprinkle with parsley.
6. Serve and enjoy!

Nutrition

Calories: 83 kcal

Cholesterol: 102.7 mg

Carbohydrates: 3 g

Protein: 6.1 g

Broccoli Chaffle with Sausage

Preparation Time: 5 minutes

Cooking Time: 18 minutes

Servings: 2

Ingredients

For chaffles:

- 1 large egg, beaten
- 1/2 cup boiled, chopped broccoli
- 1/2 cup parmesan cheese, finely grated
- A pinch of black pepper

For topping:

- 1/2 cup chicken sausage, browned and chopped
- 2 slices of Brie cheese

Directions:

1. Heat up the Chaffle maker.
2. Add all the chaffles ingredients to a small mixing bowl and combine well.
3. Set half of the batter into the Chaffle maker and Cooking for 4 minutes until golden brown.
4. Top the chaffle with warm sausage and a slice of brie cheese. Season with black pepper if desired.
5. Serve immediately and enjoy!

Nutrition:

Cal 89

Net Carbs 5.9g

Fat 6g

Protein 2g

Radishes Chaffle

Preparation Time: 5 minutes

Cooking Time: 8 minutes

Servings: 2

Ingredients:

- 1 large egg, beaten
- 1/2 cup cheddar cheese, shredded
- 1/2 tsp. baking powder
- 2 tbsp. radishes, boiled and puree
- A pinch of black pepper

Directions:

1. Heat up the Chaffle maker.
2. Attach all the ingredients to a small mixing bowl and stir until well combined.
3. Set half of the batter into the Chaffle maker and Cooking for 4 minutes until golden brown.
4. Let cool for 3 minutes to let chaffles get crispy.
5. Serve with your favorite keto dressing and enjoy!

Nutrition:

Calories: 98

Net Carb: 1.4g

Fat: 7.1g

Carbohydrates: 2.2g

Dietary Fiber: 0.8g

Savory Chaffle Sticks

Preparation Time: 5 minutes

Cooking Time: 8 minutes

Servings: 2

Ingredients:

- 1 egg, beaten
- 1/2 cup shredded parmesan cheese
- 2 tbsp. onion, browned and minced
- 1/2 tsp. paprika powder

Directions:

1. Heat up the Chaffle maker.
2. Attach all the ingredients to a small mixing bowl and combine well.
3. Set half of the batter into the Chaffle maker and Cooking for 4 minutes until golden brown.
4. Let cool for 3 minutes to let chaffles get crispy.
5. Cut the chaffles in sticks and dip into keto Tartar sauce.
6. Serve and enjoy!

Nutrition:

Cal 89

Net Carbs 5.9g

Fat 6g

Protein 2g

Beef with Cabbage Noodles

Preparation Time: 5 minutes

Cooking Time: 18 minutes

Servings: 2

Ingredients

- 4 oz. ground beef
- 1 cup chopped cabbage
- 4 oz. tomato sauce
- 1/2 tsp. minced garlic
- 1/2 cup of water
- Seasoning:
- 1/2 tbsp. coconut oil
- 1/2 tsp. salt
- 1/4 tsp. Italian seasoning
- 1/8 tsp. dried basil

Directions:

1. Take a skillet pan, place it over medium heat, add oil and when hot, add beef and Cooking for 5 minutes until nicely browned.
2. Meanwhile, prepare the cabbage and for it, slice the cabbage into thin shred.
3. When the beef has Cooked, add garlic, season with salt, basil, and Italian seasoning, stir well and continue Cooking for 3 minutes until beef has thoroughly Cooked.

4. Whisk in tomato sauce and water, stir well and bring the mixture to boil.
5. Then reduce heat to medium-low level, add cabbage, stir well until well mixed and simmer for 3 to 5 minutes until cabbage is softened, covering the pan.
6. Uncover the pan and continue simmering the beef until most of the Cooking liquid has evaporated.
7. Serve.

Nutrition: Calories: 188.5

Fats; 15.5 g

Protein: 2.5 g

Net Carb: 1

Roast Beef and Mozzarella Plate

Preparation Time: 5 minutes

Cooking Time: 0 minutes;

Servings: 2

Ingredients

- 4 slices of roast beef
- 1/2 ounce chopped lettuce
- 1 avocado, pitted
- 2 oz. mozzarella cheese, cubed
- 1/2 cup mayonnaise
- Seasoning:
- 1/4 tsp. salt
- 1/8 tsp. ground black pepper
- 2 tbsp. avocado oil

Directions:

1. Scoop out flesh from avocado and divide it evenly between two plates.
2. Add slices of roast beef, lettuce, and cheese and then sprinkle with salt and black pepper.
3. Serve with avocado oil and mayonnaise.

Nutrition:

Calories: 267.7

Fat: 24.5 g

Protein: 9.5 g

Net Carbs: 1.5 g

Fiber 2 g

Beef and Broccoli Chaffle

Preparation Time: 5 minutes

Cooking Time: 10 minutes;

Servings: 2

Ingredients

- 6 slices of beef roast, cut into strips
- 1 scallion, chopped
- 3 oz. broccoli florets, chopped
- 1 tbsp. avocado oil
- 1 tbsp. butter, unsalted

Seasoning:

- 1/4 tsp. salt
- 1/8 tsp. ground black pepper
- 1 1/2 tbsp. soy sauce
- 3 tbsp. chicken broth

Directions:

1. Take a medium skillet pan, place it over medium heat, add oil and when hot, add beef strips and Cooking for 2 minutes until hot.
2. Transfer beef to a plate, add scallion to the pan, and then add butter and Cooking for 3 minutes until tender.
3. Add remaining ingredients, stir until mixed, switch heat to the low level and simmer for 3 to 4 minutes until broccoli is tender.

4. Return beef to the pan; stir until well combined and Cooking for 1 minute.

5. Serve.

Nutrition:

Calories: 245

Fats: 15.7 g

Protein: 21.6 g

Net Carb: 1.7 g

Fiber: 1.3 g

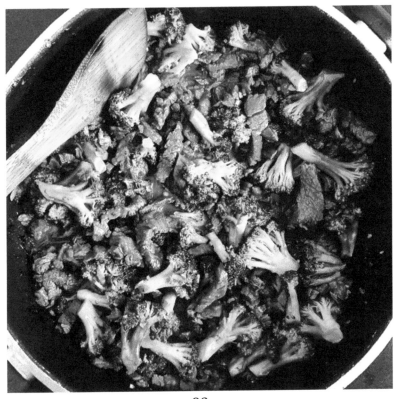

Garlic Herb Beef Roast

Preparation Time: 5 minutes

Cooking Time: 10 minutes

Servings: 2

Ingredients

- 6 slices of beef roast
- 1/2 tsp. garlic powder
- 1/3 tsp. dried thyme
- 1/4 tsp. dried rosemary
- 2 tbsp. butter, unsalted

Seasoning:

- 1/3 tsp. salt
- 1/4 tsp. ground black pepper

Directions:

1. Prepare the spice mix and for this, take a small bowl, place garlic powder, thyme, rosemary, salt, and black pepper and then stir until mixed.
2. Sprinkle spice mix on the beef roast.
3. Take a medium skillet pan, place it over medium heat, add butter and when it melts, add beef roast and then Cooking for 5 to 8 minutes until golden brown and cooked.
4. Serve.

Nutrition:

Calories: 140

Fats: 12.7 g

Protein: 5.5 g

Net Carb: 0.1 g

Fiber: 0.2 g

Sprouts Stir-fry with Kale, Broccoli, and Beef

Preparation Time: 5 minutes

Cooking Time: 8 minutes;

Servings: 2

Ingredients

- 3 slices of beef roast, chopped
- 2 oz. Brussels sprouts, halved
- 4 oz. broccoli florets
- 3 oz. kale
- 1 1/2 tbsp. butter, unsalted
- 1/8 tsp. red pepper flakes
- Seasoning:
- 1/4 tsp. garlic powder
- 1/4 tsp. salt
- 1/8 tsp. ground black pepper

Directions:

1. Take a medium skillet pan, place it over medium heat, add 3/4 tbsp. butter and when it melts, add broccoli florets and sprouts sprinkle with garlic powder, and Cooking for 2 minutes.
2. Season vegetables with salt and red pepper flakes, add chopped beef, stir until mixed and continue Cooking for 3 minutes until browned on one side.

3. Then add kale along with remaining butter, flip the vegetables and Cooking for 2 minutes until kale leaves wilts.
4. Serve.

Nutrition:

Calories: 125

Fats: 9.4 g

Protein: 4.8 g

Net Carb: 1.7 g

Fiber: 2.6 g

Beef and Vegetable Skillet

Preparation Time: 5 minutes

Cooking Time: 15 minutes

Servings: 2

Ingredients

- 3 oz. spinach, chopped
- 1/2 pound ground beef
- 2 slices of bacon, diced
- 2 oz. chopped asparagus
- Seasoning:
- 3 tbsp. coconut oil
- 2 tsp. dried thyme
- 2/3 tsp. salt
- 1/2 tsp. ground black pepper

Directions:

1. Take a skillet pan, place it over medium heat, add oil and when hot, add beef and bacon and Cooking for 5 to 7 minutes until slightly browned.
2. Then add asparagus and spinach, sprinkle with thyme, stir well and Cooking for 7 to 10 minutes until thoroughly cooked.
3. Season skillet with salt and black pepper and serve.

Nutrition:

Calories: 332.5

Fats: 26 g

Protein: 23.5 g

Net Carb: 1.5 g

Fiber: 1 g

Beef, Pepper and Green Beans Stir-fry

Preparation Time: 5 minutes;

Cooking Time: 18 minutes

Servings: 2

Ingredients

- 6 oz. ground beef
- 2 oz. chopped green bell pepper
- 4 oz. green beans
- 3 tbsp. grated cheddar cheese

Seasoning:

- 1/2 tsp. salt
- 1/4 tsp. ground black pepper
- 1/4 tsp. paprika

Directions:

1. Take a skillet pan, place it over medium heat, and add ground beef and Cooking for 4 minutes until slightly browned.
2. Then add bell pepper and green beans, season with salt, paprika, and black pepper, stir well and continue Cooking for 7 to 10 minutes until beef and vegetables have cooked through.
3. Sprinkle cheddar cheese on top, then transfer pan under the broiler and Cooking for 2 minutes until cheese has melted and the top is golden brown.
4. Serve.

Nutrition:

Calories: 282.5

Fats: 17.6 g

Protein: 26.1 g

Net Carb: 2.9 g

Fiber: 2.1 g

Cheesy Meatloaf

Preparation Time: 5 minutes

Cooking Time: 4 minutes

Servings: 2

Ingredients

- 4 oz. ground turkey
- 1 egg
- 1 tbsp. grated mozzarella cheese
- 1/4 tsp. Italian seasoning
- 1/2 tbsp. soy sauce

Seasoning:

- 1/4 tsp. salt
- 1/8 tsp. ground black pepper

Directions:

1. Take a bowl, place all the ingredients in it, and stir until mixed.
2. Take a heatproof mug, spoon in prepared mixture and microwave for 3 minutes at high heat setting until cooked.
3. When done, let meatloaf rest in the mug for 1 minute, then take it out, cut it into two slices and serve.

Nutrition:

Calories: 196.5

Fats: 13.5 g

Protein: 18.7 g

Net Carb: 18.7 g

Fiber: 0 g

Roast Beef and Vegetable Plate

Preparation Time: 10 minutes

Cooking Time: 10 minutes

Servings: 2

Ingredients

- 2 scallions, chopped in large pieces
- 1 1/2 tbsp. coconut oil
- 4 thin slices of roast beef
- 4 oz. cauliflower and broccoli mix
- 1 tbsp. butter, unsalted

Seasoning:

- 1/2 tsp. salt
- 1/3 tsp. ground black pepper
- 1 tsp. dried parsley

Directions:

1. Turn on the oven, then set it to 400 degrees F, and let it preheat.
2. Take a baking sheet, grease it with oil, place slices of roast beef on one side, and top with butter.
3. Take a separate bowl, add cauliflower and broccoli mix, add scallions, drizzle with oil, season with remaining salt and black pepper, toss until coated and then spread vegetables on the empty side of the baking sheet.
4. Bake for 5 to 7 minutes until beef is nicely browned and vegetables are tender-crisp, tossing halfway.

5. Distribute beef and vegetables between two plates and then serve.

Nutrition:

Calories: 313

Fats: 26 g

Protein: 15.6 g

Net Carb: 2.8 g

Fiber: 1.9 g

Steak and Cheese Plate

Preparation Time: 5 minutes

Cooking Time: 10 minutes

Servings: 2

Ingredients

- 1 green onion, chopped
- 2 oz. chopped lettuce
- 2 beef steaks
- 2 oz. of cheddar cheese, sliced
- 1/2 cup mayonnaise
- Seasoning:
- 1/4 tsp. salt
- 1/8 tsp. ground black pepper
- 3 tbsp. avocado oil

Directions:

1. Prepare the steak, and for this, season it with salt and black pepper.
2. Take a medium skillet pan, place it over medium heat, add oil and when hot, add seasoned steaks, and Cooking for 7 to 10 minutes until cooked to the desired level.
3. When done, distribute steaks between two plates; add scallion, lettuce, and cheese slices.
4. Drizzle with remaining oil and then serve with mayonnaise.

Nutrition:

Calories: 714

Fats: 65.3 g

Protein: 25.3 g

Net Carb: 4 g

Fiber: 5.3 g

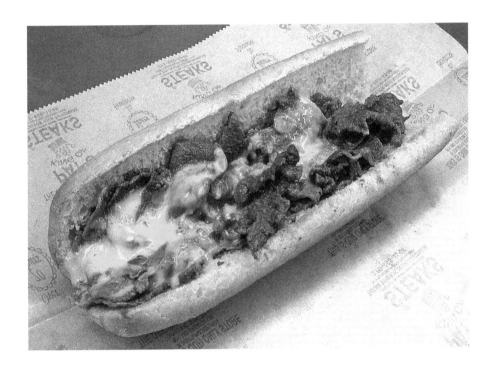

Cinnamon Chaffle Rolls

Preparation Time: 7 minutes

Cooking Time: 10 minutes

Servings: 2

Ingredients:

- 1/2 cup mozzarella cheese
- 1 tbsp. almond flour
- 1 egg
- 1 tsp. cinnamon
- 1 tsp. stevia

Cinnamon Roll Glaze

- 1 tbsp. butter
- 1 tbsp. cream cheese
- 1 tsp. cinnamon
- 1/4 tsp. vanilla extract
- 1 tbsp. coconut flour

Directions:

1. Switch on a round Chaffle maker and let it heat up.
2. In a small bowl merge together cheese, egg, flour, cinnamon powder, and stevia in a bowl.
3. Spray the round Chaffle maker with nonstick spray.
4. Pour the batter in a Chaffle maker and close the lid.
5. Close the Chaffle maker and Cooking for about 3-4 minutes.
6. Once chaffles are Cooked, remove from Maker

7. Mix together butter, cream cheese, cinnamon, vanilla and coconut flour in a bowl.

8. Spread this glaze over chaffle and roll up.

9. Serve and enjoy!

Nutrition:

Protein: 25

Fat: 69

Carbohydrates: 7

Double Chocolate Chaffles

Preparation Time: 7 minutes

Cooking Time: 5 minutes

Servings: 2

Ingredients:

- 1/4 cup unsweetened chocolate chips
- 2 tbsps. cocoa powder
- 1 cup egg whites
- 1 tsp. coffee powder
- 2 tbsps. almond flour
- 1/2 cup mozzarella cheese
- 1 tbsp. coconut milk
- 1 tsp. baking powder
- 1 tsp. stevia

Directions:

1. Switch on your Belgian chaffle maker.
2. Spray the Chaffle maker with cooking spray.
3. Set egg whites with an electric beater until fluffy and white.
4. Attach the rest of the ingredients to the egg whites and mix them again.
5. Pour batter in a greased Chaffle maker and make two fluffy chaffles.
6. Once chaffles are cooked, remove from the maker.
7. Serve with coconut cream, and berries
8. Enjoy!

Nutrition:

Protein: 52

Fat: 39

Carbohydrates: 9

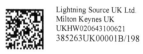